UNDERSTANDING

MELATONIN

AND BENEFITS

A Guide to Knowing its Major Targets, Focus, and Key Points for Optimal Health and Well-being

DR. LACEY MICHELLE

Disclaimer:

The information provided in this book is for general informational purposes only and is not intended as medical advice.

Readers are encouraged to consult with a qualified healthcare professional for any health concerns or questions.

Contents

About This Book

Present Melatonin Research

Current Clinical Research

Developing Subject Matter

Prospects for Melatonin Research in the Future

Wrap-Up

Comprehending Circadian Rhythms and Sleep

A vital physiological function, sleep is essential for preserving general health and well-being. It is a diverse, sophisticated process with many stages and cycles, and our circadian rhythms play a crucial role in its management. The body's internal clock, known as a circadian rhythm, controls the timing of several physiological and behavioral functions, such as the sleep-wake cycle.

the significance of rest

The human body depends on sleep to function properly. It is a dynamic process that supports multiple vital processes rather than just being a moment of idleness.

The body repairs tissue, strengthens the immune system, consolidates memories, and regulates hormones while we sleep.

 People who don't get enough sleep may suffer from a variety of detrimental effects, such as decreased cognitive function, emotional instability, and a higher chance of developing long-term health issues like obesity, diabetes, and cardiovascular illnesses.

One's physical and mental health are significantly impacted by the quantity and quality of their sleep. Adults should strive for

7-9 hours of sleep each night, though individual differences may apply.

Thus, it is crucial to comprehend and improve one's sleep habits. Sleep disorders including narcolepsy, sleep apnea, and insomnia can result from getting too little or poor-quality sleep.

The Internal Clock Of The Body

The circadian rhythm, which is the body's internal clock, regulates when different physiological activities occur.

External cues, particularly the light-dark cycle of the natural world, have an impact on this internal clock.

The body's numerous internal clocks are synchronized to the 24-hour day-night cycle by the suprachiasmatic nucleus (SCN), a small area in the hypothalamus of the brain that functions as the master pacemaker. Melatonin release is one of the hormones that the SCN controls with information gleaned from the eyes regarding light levels.

CHAPTER ONE

Melatonin's Function In Sleep Regulation

The hormone melatonin is closely linked to the body's circadian rhythms and is essential in controlling the sleep-wake cycle.

Melatonin is produced by the pineal gland, a tiny endocrine gland in the brain, mostly in reaction to lowering light levels.

The pineal gland produces more melatonin when the light fades and darkness descends, alerting the body to the impending slumber.

Melatonin is sometimes referred to as the "hormone of darkness" due to its ability to facilitate sleep and encourage relaxation.

It is an essential part of the sleep initiation process since it lowers alertness and encourages the start of sleep. Age, exposure to artificial light at night, shift work, and other variables can all affect melatonin levels and interfere with the body's normal circadian rhythms.

To fully appreciate the role that melatonin plays in controlling sleep, one must have a basic understanding of circadian rhythms and sleep. Sleep is an essential activity for preserving health and well-being, and the circadian rhythm, which regulates the body's internal clock, determines when different physiological processes occur.

The "hormone of darkness," melatonin, is essential in telling the body to get ready for sleep, and problems with melatonin production can cause problems sleeping. By gaining a comprehensive comprehension of these interrelated ideas, we can recognize how crucial melatonin supplementation is for treating sleep-related problems and enhancing sleep cycles.

Production And Regulation Of Melatonin
The intriguing hormone melatonin is essential for controlling our circadian rhythms, or sleep-wake cycles. Melatonin is mostly produced and regulated by the pineal gland, a tiny, pinecone-shaped structure found deep within the brain. The hormone in question is frequently called the "hormone of darkness" because of its strong correlation with the light-dark cycle. There is a clear rhythm to the production of melatonin, with higher amounts occurring at night and decreased levels during the day.

Methods of Melatonin Production

As the body's internal biological clock, the suprachiasmatic nucleus (SCN) in the brain sends a signal that initiates the creation of melatonin. Through the eyes, the SCN receives information about the external light-dark cycle. The sympathetic nervous system then relays this information to the pineal gland. Melatonin is produced by the pineal gland when night falls. Tryptophan is an amino acid that is transformed into serotonin, which is subsequently transformed into melatonin, in this process. To help us maintain a normal sleep-wake cycle, melatonin synthesis peaks in the middle of the night and progressively drops as daylight approaches.

Factors Influencing The Production Of Melatonin

Melatonin production is influenced by several factors. The timing and quantity of light exposure are the most important variables. Artificial light can decrease the generation of melatonin, which makes it harder for people to go to sleep. This is especially true of blue light emitted by electronic devices. On the other hand, exposure to daylight during the day aids in controlling the body's melatonin rhythm, highlighting the significance of maintaining a regular sleep pattern.

The generation of melatonin is also influenced by age. Age-related declines in melatonin levels are one of the reasons why older people frequently have altered sleep patterns.

Furthermore, melatonin production can be interfered with by several medical diseases, including sleep disorders and insomnia. The body's capacity to release melatonin at the appropriate periods can also be impacted by lifestyle choices like shift work and erratic sleep patterns.

Pineal Gland Function And Melatonin Production

The epicenter of melatonin synthesis is the pineal gland, which is found in the brain. This tiny gland, which is located deep within the brain, between the two hemispheres, is only a few millimeters in size. It is tiny, but it's incredibly important for controlling our sleep cycles and circadian rhythms.

Melatonin is produced by the pineal gland through a series of steps. It starts with tryptophan being converted to serotonin, as was previously described.

The tryptophan hydroxylase enzyme aids in this process. Then, via a sequence of enzymatic processes, serotonin is converted to melatonin. The suprachiasmatic nucleus regulates the entire process in a complex way, and light levels have a major impact on it.

Our internal biological clock and our daily exposure to light are closely linked to the generation and management of melatonin. The pineal gland is the main site of melatonin synthesis.

Our bodies' melatonin levels are influenced by several factors, including age, exposure to light, and lifestyle choices. Comprehending these ideas is crucial for handling sleep-related problems and preserving a normal circadian rhythm.

CHAPTER TWO

Using Melatonin To Promote Sleep

The pineal gland in the brain secretes melatonin, a hormone that is essential for controlling our circadian rhythm.

Melatonin supplements have been more well-known in recent years as a possible treatment for people who experience sleep difficulties, especially insomnia. Melatonin is usually over-the-counter when taken as a sleep aid, making it a desirable choice for people looking for a non-prescription way to get better sleep. Knowing the science of melatonin and how to utilize it wisely to treat sleep-related problems is crucial.

For Insomnia, Use Melatonin

A frequent sleep problem called insomnia is characterized by trouble getting to sleep, remaining asleep, or having restorative sleep. Because melatonin supplements can adjust the body's circadian clock, they are frequently thought of as a therapy option for insomnia. As day turns to night, melatonin levels normally rise in the evening, telling the body it's time to wind down and get ready for sleep.

This normal generation of melatonin may be interfered with in insomniacs, making it difficult for them to go to sleep at the appropriate time. Supplementing with melatonin can aid in improving sleep initiation and resetting the sleep-wake cycle.

Correct Dosage And Time

It's critical to utilize melatonin at the recommended dosage and time when thinking about using it as a sleep aid. Individual differences in hormone responsiveness, age, weight, and other factors can all affect the optimal dosage. In general, melatonin supplements come in a variety of shapes and sizes, including pills, candies, and liquid, with dosages ranging from one to ten milligrams or more.

The lowest effective dose is usually between 0.5 and 1 milligram, so start there and work your way up if needed. Time is also crucial, and to coincide with the body's natural melatonin release, melatonin should be taken 30 minutes to an hour before bed.

Possible Adverse Reactions And Hazards
Although melatonin is usually regarded as safe when used as directed, there are dangers and possible adverse effects. Headache, nausea, grogginess, and dizziness are a few typical adverse effects.

Usually, these effects are slight and fleeting. On the other hand, higher dosages may cause more serious adverse effects. It is advisable to seek medical advice before using melatonin supplements, particularly if you are pregnant, nursing, have underlying medical issues or are on drugs that may interact with melatonin.

Extended use of melatonin should be done with caution because the consequences of continuous supplementation over the long term are not fully established.

Furthermore, if melatonin is used improperly for an extended period, there is a potential for dependence.

It is advised to consider melatonin pills as a temporary fix for sleep problems in addition to making behavioral and lifestyle adjustments that can encourage better sleep patterns.

Melatonin is a useful supplement for treating sleeplessness and other sleep-related issues. Medication that is administered appropriately, at the right time and dosage, can assist in controlling the circadian rhythm and enhance the quality of sleep. But, anyone thinking about taking melatonin supplements has to be aware of the risks and adverse effects that may occur.

It's also a good idea to seek advice from a healthcare professional and look into alternative non-pharmacological methods of treating sleep problems.

Jet Lag And Melatonin

When travelers cross numerous time zones, they frequently experience jet lag, which throws off their circadian rhythms and can result in a variety of physical and psychological symptoms. The hormone melatonin, which is naturally produced by the pineal gland in reaction to darkness, is an important sleep-wake regulator and an effective way to lessen the effects of jet lag. This article analyzes the use of melatonin as a supplement to counteract jet lag explores its causes and symptoms, and offers ways to limit its effects.

Jet Lag Causes And Symptoms

The main cause of jet lag is a discrepancy between a person's internal body clock, or circadian rhythm, and the external time zone they are in.

The amount of time zones traveled through, the direction of travel (east or west), and a person's sensitivity all affect how severe jet lag is. The sudden change in daylight exposure can cause a variety of symptoms by interfering with the body's capacity to control sleep and waking cycles.

Fatigue, sleeplessness, trouble falling or staying asleep, irritability, mood changes, cognitive impairment, gastrointestinal issues, and a general feeling of malaise are typical signs of jet lag.

The well-being and productivity of a traveler can be greatly impacted by these symptoms while they are on the road. For those who travel frequently, jet lag poses a serious worry as it might last for several days.

Melatonin Therapy For Jet Lag

The use of melatonin pills to treat jet lag has grown in popularity. Darkness and light affect the natural hormone melatonin release, which aids in regulating the sleep-wake cycle.

Taking melatonin pills can assist in adjusting the body's internal clock to the new time zone when traveling across time zones.

When utilizing melatonin to treat jet lag, timing and dosage are crucial. Melatonin helps tell the body when it's time to go to sleep. People usually take it in the evening at the local time of their destination.

Although the dosage may vary based on personal circumstances, lesser doses (between 0.5 and 3 milligrams) are frequently advised to lessen the possibility of adverse effects.

Increased dosages might not be more beneficial and might make you drowsy when you wake up.

Before beginning melatonin supplementation, it's crucial to speak with a healthcare provider because not everyone should use it, especially if they have certain medical issues or are taking certain drugs. Melatonin is not a long-term sleep aid; rather, it should be used as a temporary measure to help with jet lag.

Techniques To Reduce Jet Lag

Although melatonin is a useful aid in jet lag management, there are a few more tactics that travelers can use to lessen its effects:

Gradual Adjustment: A few days before departure, gradually change your wake and sleep schedules to coincide with the local time. By doing this, your body adjusts to the new time zone more easily.

Keep Yourself Hydrated: It's critical to consume lots of water during your travel to prevent dehydration, which can aggravate jet lag symptoms.

Refrain from Drinking Alcohol and Caffeine: These two substances can interfere with sleep cycles.

Steer clear of these substances, especially in the few hours before bed.

Exposure to Light: Try to find natural light when you arrive at your destination during the day. Bright light exposure aids in the body's internal clock reset.

On the other hand, minimize artificial light exposure in the evening to indicate that it's time for bed.

Healthy Diet and Exercise: To improve sleep quality and general well-being, have a balanced diet and partake in mild exercise.

Napping: Take brief naps to relieve weariness, but avoid taking lengthy naps as they may disrupt your sleep at night.

While jet lag can be a difficult part of long-distance travel, there are ways to help passengers manage its effects, including taking melatonin supplements, adjusting gradually, and changing one's lifestyle. Melatonin, when administered appropriately, can help reset the body's internal clock and enhance the quality of sleep both during and after travel. To be sure it is suitable for your particular situation, it should be used sparingly and after consulting a healthcare provider.

CHAPTER THREE

Transition Work And Melatonin

Working beyond the standard 9–5 schedule is known as shift work, and it is prevalent in several sectors, including manufacturing, hospitality, transportation, and healthcare. On the other hand, it may interfere with the body's circadian cycles, which can result in a disorder called Shift Work Sleep Disorder (SWSD).

It's critical to develop measures to lessen the impacts of SWSD because it can cause sleep difficulties, decreased attentiveness, and other health problems. Melatonin supplementation is one such tactic that shift workers can take to better manage their sleep-wake cycles and general well-being.

People who work irregular hours or rotating shifts are susceptible to shift work sleep disorder, which interferes with their circadian rhythms and normal sleep cycles.

Symptoms include trouble getting asleep and staying asleep, and having restorative sleep can result from it. Those with SWSD are more likely to experience excessive sleepiness during work hours, poor cognitive function, and impaired performance.

These symptoms can be particularly problematic for those in high-alert professions like first responders and healthcare practitioners. The long-term consequences of SWSD could include an increased chance of developing chronic illnesses such as metabolic disorders, mental disorders, and cardiovascular disease.

The Use Of Melatonin By Shift Workers

The pineal gland in the brain secretes the hormone melatonin, which is principally in charge of controlling the sleep-wake cycle. Light and darkness have an impact on its secretion; melatonin levels usually rise in the evening as the body prepares for sleep. People who work shifts frequently experience sleep disturbances because they are unable to coordinate their melatonin synthesis with their changed work hours.

For shift workers, melatonin supplements can be a useful tool for modifying their circadian cycles and enhancing the quality of their sleep.

Over-the-counter melatonin supplements come in a variety of formats, including gummies, pills, and capsules. When taken as directed, melatonin can help people sleep longer and go asleep more quickly, which can lessen the negative effects of shift work on sleep patterns. Shift workers must, however, speak with a healthcare provider before beginning melatonin supplementation because timing and dosage can differ based on personal needs and schedules.

Ways To Handle Sleep During Shift Work
Apart from taking melatonin supplements, shift workers can utilize several tactics to handle their sleep and mitigate the adverse consequences of shift work disorder:

Establish a Regular Sleep routine: Try your best to stick to a regular sleep routine despite your erratic work schedule. This can assist your body in adjusting to the new schedule.

Optimize Sleep Environment: Use earplugs, blackout curtains, and a comfy mattress to create a resting environment that is conducive to slumber. Reduce the amount of noise and light pollution.

Limit Alcohol and Caffeine: Because these substances can disrupt sleep, limit your intake of alcohol and caffeine, especially in the hours before bed.

Eat Well and Stay Active: Maintaining general health and enhancing sleep can be achieved with a balanced diet and regular exercise. Avert large meals right before bed.

Make Use of Quick Power Naps: 20–30 minute power naps taken during breaks can help reduce fatigue and increase attentiveness during working hours.

Light Exposure Management: Make use of bright light exposure when working and reduce it when you're sleeping.

Adjustments to circadian rhythm can be aided by specialized light therapy equipment.

Mindfulness and Relaxation Techniques: To lower stress and enhance the quality of your sleep, try mindfulness meditation or relaxation techniques.

Seek Professional Assistance: For a thorough evaluation and tailored advice, speak with a healthcare specialist if your symptoms of SWSD are still present.

Supplementing with melatonin can help shift workers manage their sleep cycles and lessen the effects of shift work sleep disorder. To maximize sleep and general well-being in the setting of shift employment, it should be utilized in concert with other tactics. Developing a customized strategy for managing shift work sleep necessitates speaking with a healthcare professional because every person's demands are different.

Melatonin Treatment For Sleep Issues

Often called the "sleep hormone," melatonin is a hormone that is naturally present in the brain and is produced by the pineal gland. It is essential for controlling the circadian rhythm, or sleep-wake cycle, of the body. The body produces more melatonin in the evening, indicating that it is almost time for sleep.

Melatonin supplements have been more well-known in recent years as a possible treatment for a range of sleep problems and illnesses. This article explores the sorts of sleep disorders that can benefit from melatonin supplementation, how to use melatonin to treat them, and why it's important to see a doctor before taking melatonin.

Melatonin For Sleep Disorder Treatment
Supplements containing melatonin are frequently used to treat sleep disorders, especially in individuals who have trouble getting or staying asleep. The goal of melatonin supplements is to mimic and augment the body's natural melatonin production, which aids in regulating the sleep-wake cycle and enhancing the general quality of sleep.

Melatonin may be a helpful supplement for those who struggle with insomnia or other sleep-related problems, depending on their unique needs.

Melatonin primarily works by interacting with brain receptors that aid in the initiation of sleep. Melatonin, when supplemented, can improve the duration and quality of sleep as well as shorten the time it takes to fall asleep (sleep onset latency). As it can assist in realigning their internal body clock with their preferred sleep pattern, it is especially beneficial for people with circadian rhythm abnormalities, such as jet lag or shift work-related sleep issues.

Melatonin comes in several forms, such as liquid solutions, gummies, tablets, and capsules. The right decision for an individual's particular sleep condition, age, and general health will determine the dosages and types that are available. It is important to remember that melatonin's benefits can differ from person to person and that there is no one-size-fits-all answer.

Sleep Disorders for Which Melatonin May Be Beneficial

Supplementing with melatonin may be beneficial for several diseases including sleep disturbances. These consist of:

Primary insomniacs may find melatonin to be beneficial, particularly if they have trouble falling asleep. It can shorten the period needed to fall asleep, encouraging a better night's sleep.

Delayed Sleep-Wake Phase condition (DSWPD): This circadian rhythm condition causes a person's natural sleep-wake cycle to be delayed, which makes it difficult for them to go to sleep at night and wake up in the morning. It is possible to change this delayed cycle earlier with melatonin, which will facilitate going to sleep and waking up at preferred times.

Jet Lag: The body's internal clock can fall out of sync with the local time when traversing various time zones. Melatonin pills might help you get used to the new time zone faster and lessen jet lag symptoms.

Shift Work Sleep Disorder: It might be difficult for people to have a normal sleep schedule when they work night or irregular shifts. Melatonin can help people sleep better and adjust to their new work schedules.

Children's sleep disturbances: When children struggle to fall asleep due to sleep disorders like night terrors, melatonin supplements may be prescribed. Nonetheless, it's vital to speak with a pediatrician before giving melatonin to kids.

aging-Related Sleep Changes: Melatonin production can decline with aging, which can cause sleep problems. Supplementing with melatonin may benefit elderly people who have trouble sleeping.

Speaking With A Medical Professional

A healthcare provider, such as a primary care physician or a sleep expert, should be consulted before beginning melatonin supplementation to treat a sleep disturbance. This is an important step for a few reasons:

Precise Diagnosis: The underlying reason for the sleep disturbance can be precisely identified by a medical practitioner. Different treatment modalities may be needed for various sleep problems.

Tailored therapy Plan: Considering each patient's unique requirements and medical background, medical experts can offer tailored advice on melatonin dosage, timing, and therapy duration.

Safety and Adverse Effects: Supplementing with melatonin may have adverse effects and interactions with other medications just like taking any other medication. A medical expert can evaluate any dangers and offer advice on appropriate use.

Progress tracking: Scheduling routine appointments with a medical practitioner enables the tracking of melatonin supplementation's efficacy and the making of any required alterations to the treatment regimen.

When used as a therapeutic technique for different types of sleep disorders, melatonin can help people sleep better and feel better overall. To guarantee safe and efficient usage and to meet the unique needs of every person with a sleep disturbance, it should, nevertheless, be used under the supervision of a healthcare provider.

Melatonin can be a useful supplement to a comprehensive management strategy for sleep disorders and disturbances when taken appropriately.

CHAPTER FOUR

Melatonin And Additional Health Advantages

The pineal gland in the brain naturally produces melatonin, a hormone well recognized for controlling sleep-wake cycles. Beyond its effects on sleep, melatonin has been shown to have several additional health benefits. The antioxidant qualities of melatonin are one of its noteworthy features, which add to its complex function in enhancing general well-being.

Melatonin's Antioxidant Properties

Because melatonin is a strong antioxidant, it can counteract the body's production of dangerous chemicals known as free radicals. Unstable molecules known as free radicals have the potential to harm cells and have a role in several health problems, such as aging and chronic illnesses. By scavenging these free radicals, melatonin helps shield DNA and cells from oxidative stress.

Melatonin's capacity to readily pass through cell membranes and enter many cellular compartments, including the nucleus, is one of its special qualities as an antioxidant.

This makes it possible for melatonin to shield DNA and vital biological components, lowering the possibility of DNA damage and mutations. Melatonin may be a viable treatment option for disorders and diseases linked to oxidative stress because of its antioxidant qualities.

The anti-oxidant qualities of melatonin may play a role in the management and prevention of diseases like heart disease, Parkinson's disease, and Alzheimer's disease, as well as some forms of cancer. Melatonin may be very helpful in maintaining general health and may delay the onset of age-related illnesses by lowering inflammation and oxidative damage.

Potential Uses Not Just For Sleep

Although controlling the circadian clock and enhancing the quality of sleep are melatonin's main functions, the hormone has been shown to provide benefits in several other areas of health. Melatonin pills, for example, are frequently used to treat jet lag symptoms and shift work-related sleep problems. People can more easily adjust to different time zones and work schedules thanks to melatonin's capacity to change the internal body clock.

Additionally, melatonin has demonstrated promise in the treatment of mood disorders, especially in those with seasonal affective disorder (SAD) and some types of depression. Its effects on serotonin synthesis and sleep-wake cycle management may help stabilize mood and enhance mental wellness.

Furthermore, melatonin's ability to enhance fertility and reproductive health has been investigated. According to some research, melatonin may improve the quality of sperm and eggs, which may be helpful for infertile couples.

Studies on melatonin's effects on the immune system have shown that it can lower inflammation and improve immunological function. This has consequences for immunological dysregulation-related disorders such as autoimmune illnesses.

The many health benefits of melatonin are still being thoroughly studied. Researchers are looking into its possible uses for a variety of ailments, including neuroprotection, COVID-19 treatment, and cancer management and prevention.

Research is still being done to determine how melatonin can affect immune response and possibly help treat viral infections like COVID-19. In some circumstances, its anti-inflammatory and antioxidant qualities might help lessen the intensity of symptoms and encourage healing.

Researchers are also very interested in melatonin's ability to slow down aging and mitigate age-related disorders, especially as the aging population continues to rise. Research is still being done on the effects of melatonin administration on longevity, cognitive function, and general quality of life.

Even though melatonin's function in controlling sleep is well known, there is still much to learn about this intriguing substance due to its antioxidant qualities and wide range of potential uses in health and wellbeing. Melatonin may find more uses in medicine and contribute to better health and well-being in a range of circumstances as our knowledge of its many advantages grows.

Selecting An Appropriate Melatonin Supplement

It's crucial to do your research before choosing a melatonin supplement to make sure you're getting the best one for your needs. Our sleep-wake cycle is mostly regulated by the hormone melatonin, which is naturally produced by the pineal gland in the brain. On the other hand, some people might require melatonin supplements to treat jet lag, sleep difficulties, or other conditions that throw off their circadian cycle. One needs to consider several important variables to make an informed decision.

Different Melatonin Supplement Types
There are many different forms of melatonin supplements on the market, such as tablets, capsules, gummies, and even liquids. Selecting the right kind of supplement frequently comes down to personal needs and tastes.

For example, you may prefer melatonin gummies or a liquid form if you have trouble swallowing pills. The chosen form's bioavailability and absorption must be taken into account, though. For people looking for speedy results, sublingual (dissolvable under the tongue) melatonin may be absorbed more quickly than conventional oral tablets.

Moreover, there are melatonin pills with an extended-release that are made to replicate the body's natural melatonin production by releasing melatonin gradually throughout the night.

This may be helpful for people who experience persistent sleep difficulties. Furthermore, the efficacy of certain melatonin supplements may be increased when mixed with other components that promote sleep, such as chamomile or valerian root.

Your unique sleep requirements and preferences should be taken into consideration while selecting the right kind of melatonin supplement.

Aspects Of Purity And Quality To Consider

Pure and high-quality ingredients are crucial when selecting a melatonin supplement. Between brands and manufacturers, melatonin products might differ greatly in terms of strength and purity.

Take into account the following to make sure you are purchasing a high-quality product:

Third-party testing: To confirm a product's potency and purity, look for tests conducted by trustworthy, independent laboratories. By doing this, it is made sure that the product's contents and its label match.

Accurate dosage: Verify that the melatonin dosage is appropriate for your needs.

Although the usual dosage range is 1 to 10 milligrams, certain people may respond better to lesser amounts.

Lack of fillers and additives: Check the ingredient list to be sure there aren't any extraneous fillers or additives that could reduce melatonin's effectiveness or produce negative side effects.

Manufacturing standards: To assist in guaranteeing the product's quality and consistency, choose goods from producers who adhere to Good Manufacturing Practices (GMP).

The synthetic form of melatonin is the same as the melatonin produced by the human body and is generally more dependable and consistent in terms of purity.

Rules And Safety Instructions

Melatonin supplements are easily accessible because they are sold over-the-counter in many countries. This does not imply that they are risk- or side-effect-free, though. It's critical to understand the following rules and principles about safety:

Speak with a healthcare provider: It's essential to speak with a healthcare provider before beginning melatonin supplementation, particularly if you have any underlying medical concerns, are pregnant or nursing, or are taking medication.

A healthcare provider can assist in determining the proper dosage and timing of melatonin because it may interfere with certain medications and medical conditions.

Age and dosage considerations: Although large doses and prolonged usage of melatonin supplements may result in negative consequences, they are usually regarded as safe for short-term use. If necessary, dosages should be adjusted based on age, giving adults higher doses and children lower ones.

Timing: To align with your circadian cycle, melatonin should be taken at the appropriate time. If you take it too soon, it may interfere with your regular sleep-wake pattern.

Although melatonin is generally well accepted, adverse effects may manifest as headaches, dizziness, and blood pressure fluctuations.

It is imperative to be cognizant of these possible adverse consequences.

Selecting the best melatonin supplement requires taking into account your needs and preferences, as well as guaranteeing the product's quality and purity through independent testing, compliance with production standards, and observance of safety directives and laws. Melatonin supplements can be a useful tool for treating circadian rhythm abnormalities and promoting better sleep if used with caution.

CHAPTER FIVE

Risks And Adverse Reactions

The pineal gland in the brain secretes the hormone melatonin, which is essential for controlling the cycle of sleep and wakefulness.

Additionally, it comes in a variety of supplement forms, including gummies, tablets, and capsules. Although melatonin supplements are typically regarded as safe when taken for a brief period, consumers should be informed of the dangers and possible adverse effects. Comprehending these hazards and adverse reactions is vital to create knowledgeable choices regarding melatonin ingestion.

Potential Adverse Reactions With Melatonin

Supplements containing melatonin are frequently used to treat sleep-related conditions like jet lag and insomnia. Though these are usually moderate, they can have adverse effects just like any other prescription or supplement. Symptoms of melatonin supplementation that are frequently experienced include headache, nausea, and tiredness.

It's important to remember that these adverse effects usually pass quickly as the body becomes used to the supplement.

More severe adverse effects, like vivid dreams, nightmares, or even an aggravation of pre-existing sleep disorders, may occasionally be experienced by people. Although less frequent, some users may find these effects upsetting. Melatonin users should stop using the drug and seek medical advice if they encounter strange or severe side effects.

Extended Safety Issues

The safety of melatonin over the long term is one of the main issues surrounding its use. Since there has been little research on the long-term use of melatonin supplements, it is unknown what dangers might arise from continued use. It's critical to understand that melatonin is meant to be used as a short-term, infrequent sleep aid; prolonged use is not advised.

Furthermore, prolonged use of melatonin supplements may interfere with the body's normal synthesis of the hormone, which could result in a decrease in endogenous melatonin production. This may eventually cause the body to become dependent on outside supplements to sustain a normal sleep-wake cycle. When thinking about using melatonin for an extended period, people should speak with a healthcare professional to assess the advantages and disadvantages and look into other options for treating sleep issues.

Particular Attention To Some Groups

Not everyone should take melatonin supplements, and there are certain things to think about for particular demographics. There is little data on the safety of melatonin supplements in pregnant and lactating women, therefore they should use caution when using them.

Generally speaking, before using melatonin, those who are pregnant or nursing should speak with a healthcare provider.

Additionally, the demands and reactions of children and teenagers to melatonin may differ. Since the long-term effects of melatonin supplements on development are unknown, its usage in this age range should be under the guidance of a healthcare professional.

Before using melatonin, anyone with underlying medical conditions—especially those with autoimmune illnesses, epilepsy, or drugs that influence the immune system or blood clotting—should speak with a healthcare provider.

It may not be a good idea to use melatonin in conjunction with current medical conditions or treatments because it may interfere with some drugs.

In the short term, melatonin supplements may be a useful tool for treating sleep-related problems, but it's important to be aware of the risks and adverse effects. Caution should be exercised when using for an extended period, and particular populations should receive extra attention. People should speak with a healthcare professional before starting melatonin supplements to make sure it is safe and appropriate for their unique situation.

Melatonin In Combination With Other Methods

Melatonin supplementation can be a useful tool for treating sleep problems, but it works best when combined with other strategies. Melatonin's effectiveness varies from person to person, and in certain cases, it might not be enough to treat sleep issues on its own. Enhancing sleep quality can be accomplished more thoroughly and uniquely by combining melatonin with other methods.

Way Of Living And Sleep Hygiene

Our sleep patterns are greatly influenced by our lifestyle choices and sleep hygiene practices. Supplementing with melatonin can be made much more effective by implementing appropriate sleep habits. Better sleep can be facilitated by a balanced diet, frequent exercise, and a regular sleep pattern. Reducing alcohol and caffeine consumption can also help you get a better night's sleep, particularly in the hours before bed. Melatonin's ability to promote sleep can also be strengthened by creating a cozy sleeping environment, such as a cool, dark, and quiet room.

Insomnia Treatment with Cognitive Behavioral Therapy (CBT-I)

Melatonin supplements can be used in conjunction with a well-researched treatment strategy called Cognitive Behavioral Therapy for Insomnia (CBT-I).

The goal of CBT-I is to alter the mental processes and behaviors that lead to insomnia. It frequently consists of methods for dealing with the tension and worry that can prevent you from falling asleep.

CBT-I can assist people in changing their negative sleep-related attitudes and forming improved sleep habits. CBT-I can offer a comprehensive treatment for chronic insomnia by treating the psychological and physiological components of sleep disorders when paired with melatonin.

Melatonin And Medication

Prescription medicine may be necessary for people who experience significant sleep disruptions in certain situations. Usually, people who have not reacted well to previous therapies are the ones prescribed these drugs. One way to maximize the benefits of pharmaceutical sleep aids while reducing adverse effects is to take melatonin in addition to them.

Benzodiazepines are a class of drugs that are frequently taken in conjunction with melatonin; they are depressants of the central nervous system. Benzodiazepines can lessen anxiety and encourage relaxation when used with melatonin, which may enhance the quality of sleep.

 However, because of their potential for reliance and negative effects, these drugs must be used under the supervision of a healthcare provider.

Medications classified as non-benzodiazepine hypnotics, such as zolpidem and eszopiclone, can also be taken in combination with melatonin.

The purpose of these medications is to aid in the start and maintenance of sleep. Together with melatonin, they can provide a more well-rounded treatment for insomnia by addressing the time and general quality of sleep.

It's crucial to remember that taking melatonin with prescription drugs should always be under a doctor's supervision because drug interactions can have unanticipated effects.

When all other options have failed, this strategy should be considered a last resort and applied with caution.

Even while melatonin supplements can be a useful tool for enhancing sleep, they work best when paired with other strategies.

When combined with melatonin, supplementary techniques such as CBT-I, medicine, and lifestyle and sleep hygiene can offer a more holistic solution for people with sleep difficulties. To guarantee the greatest potential outcome for each patient, the combination of tactics to be used should ultimately be customized and directed by a healthcare practitioner.

CHAPTER SIX

Individual Narratives And Achievements

The pineal gland in the brain is the primary source of melatonin, a hormone that the body naturally produces and which is essential for controlling our circadian rhythm. Although melatonin pills are frequently used to treat sleep-related problems, firsthand accounts and success stories highlight the hormone's potential benefits for enhancing sleep quality and treating a range of sleep disorders.

Actual Testimonials

Testimonials from real people are a great resource for anyone looking for answers to their sleep issues. Numerous individuals have discussed their experiences with melatonin tablets, frequently highlighting the improvements in their sleep patterns that they have experienced. These anecdotes frequently center on people who have battled jet lag, sleeplessness, or other sleep-related issues.

Those who use melatonin supplements report improved sleep after experiencing sleep problems, such as trouble getting or staying asleep. Melatonin can assist folks who suffer from insomnia to fall asleep faster and have better-quality sleep overall. Some people have discovered that using melatonin supplements lessens their need for other sleep aids or prescription drugs because they provide a non-habit-forming alternative.

Jet lag sufferers have also reported benefits from melatonin.

Melatonin pills can help acclimate to the local schedule, allowing for a smoother transfer and lessening the impacts of jet lag, according to travelers who need to shift to new time zones.

Melatonin pills have proven to be a helpful tool for shift workers who struggle with irregular sleep habits and need time to adjust to their shifting work schedules. These people can maintain a better quality of sleep, which is essential for general well-being, by controlling their sleep-wake cycle.

Motivating Testimonials Of Better Sleep

Positive reports of better sleep achieved with melatonin tablets are common. People have talked about how melatonin has helped them feel in control of their sleep schedules and has made it possible for them to have more peaceful nights. Melatonin has been adopted by those who just wish to improve the quality of their sleep, in addition to treating specific sleep-related issues.

It is crucial to remember that while melatonin can be quite beneficial for many people, each person's reaction is unique. Some people could need melatonin supplements in different amounts or formats, like liquid or time-release tablets. The effectiveness of melatonin supplements may also be influenced by other elements including nutrition, lifestyle, and general health.

Individuals' sleep patterns and quality can be positively impacted by melatonin supplementation, as demonstrated by success stories and personal experiences. These testimonies demonstrate how adaptable melatonin is and how it can help people who are looking for better sleep, whether they are suffering from jet lag, insomnia, shift work, or other conditions. To guarantee melatonin is used safely and effectively, as with any supplement or prescription, speak with a healthcare provider before adding it to your sleep management plan.

CHAPTER SEVEN

The Prospects For Melatonin Studies

The pineal gland secretes the hormone melatonin, which has long been linked to controlling circadian rhythms and the sleep-wake cycle. Its function goes well beyond that of a simple sleep aid, though. Melatonin has several potential uses, and future studies should reveal these uses in a variety of contexts. Its complex mechanics are being clarified and its horizon is being expanded by ongoing investigations.

Current Research And Emerging Discoveries

Recent studies are revealing melatonin's profound influence on human health. Research is looking into how it affects cardiovascular health, the immune system, and possibly the prevention of cancer. The capacity of melatonin to shield cells from oxidative damage and maybe lower the risk of certain diseases has drawn attention to the substance's antioxidant qualities. Its neuroprotective role, which may be important in the treatment of neurodegenerative diseases including Alzheimer's and Parkinson's disease, is also shown by emerging research.

Additionally, research on melatonin's relationship with the gut microbiota is also ongoing. Melatonin and gut health have been related in recent research, which may have consequences for diseases including inflammatory bowel disease and irritable bowel syndrome. Melatonin plays an increasingly important role in preserving a healthy equilibrium within this complex ecosystem as our understanding of the gut-brain relationship deepens.

Prospective Developments And Uses

Numerous intriguing potential discoveries in melatonin research exist. Future uses for melatonin supplements may include mental health issues in addition to sleep disorders, jet lag, and shift work, which have already made them popular. Melatonin may help control anxiety and depression, according to certain research. Should additional investigation validate these assertions, it might present a fresh method for addressing these prevalent mental health issues.

Furthermore, there is research on how melatonin affects body weight and metabolism. Melatonin may be used in the future to treat metabolic problems including obesity. It might be used in conjunction with other weight-management techniques, particularly for people who are experiencing circadian rhythm disruption—a prevalent problem in contemporary culture.

What Melatonin Has In Store

It is impossible to ignore the possibility of novel cures and treatments as melatonin research advances. Exploring the impact of melatonin on longevity and aging is yet another uncharted territory. One area of promising research is whether melatonin can slow down the aging process and increase longevity.

The expanding field of customized medicine and melatonin's future are intertwined. It might soon be possible to customize melatonin administration to a person's unique circadian rhythm and medical requirements. This targeted method may improve melatonin's effectiveness in treating mental health issues, sleep difficulties, and other conditions.

Conclusion

Research on melatonin has a bright future ahead of it. Its involvement in various facets of human health, such as the immune system and the gut-brain link, is becoming clearer via ongoing research. Melatonin can address a wide range of ailments, from weight to mental health. The advancements in its uses are similarly promising.

Melatonin has a wide range of applications as we learn more about its functions and effects. Melatonin offers novel treatments for a range of health issues, and it may be a key factor in determining the direction of health and medicine in the future. We should soon be able to fully realize the benefits of melatonin and its profound effects on human health and well-being through more investigation and study.